For Kicks and Giggles

LAUGHING THROUGH PREGNANCY'S QUIRKIEST MOMENTS

Lighthearted, relatable, and humorous short stories that women can have a (pregnant) belly laugh at.

JULIA DUFFY

ISBN-13: 9781234567890

ISBN-10: 1477123456

Library of Congress Control Number: 2018675309

Printed in the United States of America

Table of Contents

Introduction

In the grand adventure of life, few journeys are as transformative and profound as the path to parenthood. From the moment those two little lines appear on the pregnancy test; your world is irrevocably altered. Welcome to "For Kicks and Giggles: Laughing Through Pregnancy's Quirkiest Moments," a heartfelt and candid exploration of the incredible journey that is pregnancy. Within these pages, we will embark on a captivating voyage offering a unique lens into the exhilarating, sometimes bewildering, and often humorous world of expecting a baby.

Prologue

The Prelude to Parenthood

In the hushed moments before parenthood, there exists a world of anticipation and wonder. It's a time of dreams, laughter, and preparation for the grand adventure ahead. The journey begins not at birth but with the first flutter of life, an invitation to enter a realm where every day brings a new surprise, a new lesson, and often, a new reason to chuckle. As you embark on this rollercoaster ride, remember that humor is your trusty companion. From the quirks of maternity fashion to the unsolicited advice that flows like a river, this book unfolds a tale of parenthood through the lens of laughter. It's a reminder that even in the midst of challenges and sleepless nights, there's always room for a good laugh. So, fasten your seatbelt and get ready for a journey filled with humor, heart, and the beautiful chaos of parenthood.

Chapter 1

Cravings and Food Aversions: A Culinary Adventure

Ah, the mystical realm of pregnancy cravings and food aversions. It's like embarking on a gastronomic journey where your taste buds become the navigators and your fridge transforms into a treasure chest of delights and, well, questionable choices.

Let's paint a pretty little picture: it's 2 AM, and you're suddenly possessed by the idea of pickle-flavored caramel ice cream. It's as if your brain has merged the contents of the pantry and the fridge into an unholy alliance, and your cravings are the bizarre offspring. You tiptoe to the kitchen, illuminated only by the light of the fridge, and stare at the pickles, the caramel sauce, and the vanilla ice cream like a mad scientist pondering her creation.

But let's not forget the ever-so-loyal food aversions. Suddenly, the sight and smell of your once-beloved coffee trigger an almost superhero-like ability to detect the faintest whiff from miles away. Your spouse innocently brews a cup in the next room, and you burst through the door, nostrils flaring, like a bloodhound on a caffeine-related mission. It's a peculiar dance of love and betrayal where your taste buds turn into real biatches.

And then there's the classic scenario of craving something that's just impossible to acquire. You have a hankering for a double cheeseburger from a specific fast-food joint located three states away. You'd consider a road trip if it weren't for the fact that you're currently lounging on the couch, having mastered the art of rolling to your side without losing your equilibrium.

Let's not forget the odd combinations. Suddenly, your snack of choice is peanut butter and pickles, and your significant other looks at you like you've just discovered a new planet. You try to explain that it's a gourmet masterpiece that only pregnancy can truly appreciate, but their doubtful gaze remains.

Of course, these cravings and aversions are complete a-holes and have no respect for the time of day. Breakfast foods become dinner staples, and dinner becomes a parade of breakfast cereals. You stare at your plate, wondering how it came to this—a symphony of flavors that Mozart himself would never have composed.

But hey, these cravings and aversions come with their own kind of magic. They remind you that you're on a unique journey, one where your body is working tirelessly to create a new life. So, whether you're munching on pickles and ice cream at dawn or suddenly declaring a truce with broccoli, know that you're not alone in this culinary adventure. Someday, you'll look back and chuckle at the time you waged a war with the pantry, armed with nothing but pickled onions and a bag of marshmallows.

Chapter 2

Baby Brain Moments: When Your Brain Goes on Maternity Leave Too

The concept of "baby brain" may sound like a fairy tale told among circles of expectant mothers, but anyone who's been through the rollercoaster of pregnancy knows it's all too real. It's like your brain, in solidarity with your feet, decides to swell up and temporarily loses its ability to function in familiar ways. Like your brain has decided to take a little vacation while your body embarks on the adventure of a lifetime.

Remember the time you decided to go for a jog, put on your detective hat, and embarked on an epic quest to find your missing sneakers? You turned your house upside down, inside out, and practically tore your hair out in frustration. But little did you know, the real comedy was happening right under your nose. Literally.

There you were, all geared up to embrace the world of fitness, ready to take to the pavement and sweat out the pregnancy cravings. You knew it was a challenge, but you were determined. Step one: locate those elusive sneakers.

You started in the living room, thinking, "Maybe I kicked them under the sofa." You crouched, contorted, and contended with dust bunnies, but all you found were a couple of lost toys and some spare change. Shit, and now you're stuck on the floor.

Undeterred, you moved to the bedroom, convinced that your sneakers had somehow migrated there. You flipped cushions, ransacked your closet, and briefly considered posting to social media, convinced you'd forgotten lending them out to a friend. But no sneakers. Only more frustration.

Finally, after an exhaustive house-wide search, you gave up. You couldn't hold back the tears any longer. The sheer ridiculousness of it all pushed you to the edge, and you sat down on the stairs, ready to weep for your lost jog.

As you sat there, despairing of your shoeless fate, you looked down at your swollen feet, which were nestled comfortably inside... your sneakers. Yep, the very ones you'd been desperately hunting down for the past half-hour. They hadn't gone on a walkabout; they'd been faithfully waiting for you all along. But when the eff did you put them on in the first place?

Cue the laughter, or in your case, the mix of hysterical giggles, tears, and sighs of relief. How could you have missed something so obvious? It's as if your sneakers decided to play a little prank on you, proving that pregnancy brain can lead to moments of hilarity even in the midst of frustration.

I've said it once, and I'll say it again: You. Are. Not. Alone. (Spoiler alert: sometimes baby brain never goes away.) Pregnancy has its unique way of keeping you on your toes, even when those toes are already inside your shoes.

Chapter 3

Baby Names and Gender Predictions:
The Great Debate

Choosing a name for your baby is like embarking on a quest to find the perfect title for a novel. It's a mix of excitement, creativity, and a touch of absurdity. And while you're at it, you'll also discover that everyone around you has suddenly transformed into a baby name expert and gender prediction guru.

The Name Game: Classic vs. Trending Celeb Baby Names

You and your partner sit down with a baby name book that's thicker than a phone directory. Classic names like Emily, James, and Sophia make the list, and you imagine your child as a timeless figure, perhaps destined to write poetry or lead a nation.

But then, in a moment of whimsy, you throw in a wildcard like "Moon Unit." For a moment you let your mind wander and even begin to envision the nights ahead gazing up at the night sky with your little sidekick, Moonie.

As you share your name ideas with friends and family, you're met with a range of reactions. Some nod approvingly at the classics, while others give you puzzled looks when "Apple" enters the conversation. You find humor in their bewildered expressions, secretly pleased that you've added a dash of eccentricity to the mix.

The Expert Gender Predictors:

As your belly grows, so does the collective wisdom of your friends, family, and even acquaintances when it comes to predicting your baby's gender. Suddenly, your cravings become the oracle of truth. If you crave rotisserie chicken, it's definitely a boy, but if it's cupcakes, it's undoubtedly a girl.

You chuckle as you contemplate the fact that your baby's gender hinges on whether you prefer salty or sweet snacks. But you humor your well-meaning advisors, secretly enjoying the suspense of keeping the true gender a mystery.

Then come the dreams. Your aunt swears that her dream about flying pink elephants the night before your baby shower is a sure sign that you're having a girl. You nod and smile, mentally filing her dream interpretation alongside the Moxie CrimeFighter name suggestion.

And let's not forget the age-old gender prediction legends. The neighbor who swears that if your belly sits high, it's a girl, but if it's low, it's a boy. You've now become the subject of a neighborhood betting pool, with odds shifting based on the height of your bump.

The Ultimate Reveal: Laughing All the Way
In the end, whether you choose a classic name or opt for something as whimsical as "Cricket Pearl," and whether your cravings lean towards peanut butter or raspberry licorice, one thing is certain: the joy and laughter that come with the baby naming and gender prediction saga are priceless.

You chuckle at the well-intentioned advice-givers and savor the moments of shared laughter as you navigate this delightful journey into parenthood. So, embrace the creativity, enjoy the camaraderie, and get ready for the grand reveal when your baby finally makes their debut, regardless of whether they arrive with a classic name, or a name destined for the tabloids.

Chapter 4

Sleep Struggles: The Comedy of Midnight Maneuvers

Pregnancy, they say, is like training for a marathon. You're preparing for those sleepless nights ahead with nightly rehearsals in the art of sleep struggles. You don't just sleep; you engage in a highly choreographed performance. It's a mix of acrobatics, ninja moves, and bladder ballet, and well… it's ridiculous.

The 12-Step Pillow Fort

First, let's talk about the mystical 12-step pillow fortress. This intricate arrangement involves strategically placing pillows around your body: under your belly, between your knees, and sometimes even over your head if you're feeling adventurous. Your partner watches in awe as you build this monument to comfort.

But here's the twist: every time you need to turn over (which happens roughly every 10 minutes because one of your limbs will undoubtably betray you and fall asleep for no reason), you must deconstruct and then rebuild this fortress. It's like a nightly ritual that involves more grunt work than a CrossFit session.

Some nights, you even find yourself debating the structural integrity of your pillow fort. Will it support you through the night, or will it crumble like a house of cards? Spoiler alert: It usually crumbles, and you end up wrestling with your pillows more than a WWE champion.

The Bladder's Revenge

Just when you've finally achieved a position of perfect comfort, the bladder decides it's time for revenge. It doesn't matter that you've only just drained the ol' gal; she's back for another round.

Maybe if you just lay here long enough, she'll get tired of playing these surprise attacks on your tranquility. But alas, it's a battle of wills, and that bladder has an uncanny ability to summon its forces whenever it pleases.

Is this what they meant by "sleepless nights" in the parenting brochures? Perhaps this is all a conspiracy orchestrated by the adult diaper industry, secretly plotting to make you a lifelong customer. You contemplate the monthly subscription box.

And so, you embark on yet another nocturnal mission, navigating the obstacle course of squeaky floors, dimly lit hallways, and the eternal struggle between sleep and nature's call. Back to navigating the obstacle course of your 12-step pillow fort once more.

Chapter 5

Maternity Fashion Follies: Rocking the Potato Sack Chic

Pregnancy also brings many changes, including a sudden shift in your relationship with your closet. Those stylish skinny jeans and tailored blouses start to look more like medieval torture devices than fashion statements. Hard no. Welcome to the world of maternity fashion follies, where comfort often takes precedence over style, and you become a connoisseur of "potato sack chic."

Potato Sack Chic: The Comfy Revolution

Remember when you used to spend hours carefully selecting the perfect outfit for the day? Now, the criterion is simple: Will it fit over your belly without inducing suffocation? If yes, it's a winner. The potato sack chic look becomes your go-to style.

You find yourself raiding the "comfy" section of the department store, gravitating toward anything that resembles a potato sack with leg holes. Maxi dresses become your BFFs. Your closet is filled with an assortment of flowy, oversized garments in shades that can only be described as "variations of black" to hide potential stains from unpredictable cravings.

Accessories and Footwear: The Final Frontier
As your belly continues its remarkable expansion, you find yourself staring down the challenges of two crucial aspects of fashion: footwear and accessories. Suddenly, the simple act of bending over to tie your shoes feels like you've signed up for an Olympic gymnastics routine. You debate between investing in a shoehorn the size of a canoe paddle or just wholeheartedly embracing the "slip-on shoes only" look for the foreseeable future.

And then there are the accessories. Scarves, once fashion statements, now double as makeshift bibs, ready to catch crumbs from your impromptu midnight snack sessions. Who knew your neckwear would moonlight as a crumb-catcher?

So, whether you're waddling around in slip-on shoes or mastering the art of accessorizing, remember that pregnancy fashion isn't just about style; it's about survival. It's about finding inventive ways to navigate the final frontier of expanding waistlines and limited mobility, all while looking fabulous in the process. Who said pregnancy couldn't be fashion forward?

In the Company of Comrades
The beauty of maternity fashion initiates a bond with other pregnant individuals over the shared

experience of sacrificing style for comfort. There's camaraderie in knowing that your fellow maternity fashionistas are also embracing potato sack chic.

In the end, it's all a testament to your adaptability and resourcefulness during pregnancy. It's a reminder that fashion rules can be rewritten, and that comfort can indeed be fashionable. So, don't be afraid to rock that oversized T-shirt, embrace the flowy maxi dresses, and wear your potato sack chic badge with pride, sista.

Chapter 6

Unsolicited Advice: The Great Parade of Wisdom

Pregnancy seems to have a magical power, turning perfect strangers into self-appointed life coaches. It's like wearing a neon sign that screams, "Tell me what to do!" Welcome to the world of unsolicited advice, where you'll meet a cast of characters who just can't resist sharing their pearls of wisdom. *Insert eye roll*

The Supermarket Saga

Picture this: You, a determined and heavily pregnant superhero, have embarked on a mission to conquer the treacherous terrain of grocery shopping. You navigate the aisles with the grace of a sumo wrestler in a ballet recital, breathing heavily with every step.

Finally, you reach the self-checkout line, your sanctuary, and the finish line of your expedition. You're just trying to scan your pickles (because cravings wait for no one) when a well-meaning but bewildered fellow shopper eyes you with concern.

They lean in, and in their most serious "I'm-ready-to-save-the-day" tone, they ask, "Are you in labor?"

You pause, scanning their face for any sign of jest. Surely, they're kidding, right? You look down at your belly, which, though impressive, is not yet the size of a hot air balloon. Then, you flash a grin and respond with a hint of playful sarcasm, "Oh, no, not quite. I've got three more months of this glorious adventure!"

The would-be savior blinks in surprise. It turns out that your pregnant superpowers include summoning comedic relief even in the most unexpected situations. Who knew that growing a tiny human could be so entertaining?

The Queue Consultant

While waiting in line at the post office, you strike up a conversation with a friendly fellow queue mate. You mention your upcoming due date, and suddenly, you're bombarded with stories of their aunt's cousin's friend who had an unusual pregnancy complication. They assure you that it's vital to keep an eye out for it.

You smile, thinking about the statistical improbability of facing the same scenario. But you humor them, wondering if you should start an unsolicited advice bingo card.

Aunt's cousin's friend's story—check.

The Social Media Guru

Ah, the age of social media—the perfect platform to share life's milestones with friends, family, and sometimes complete strangers. Your pregnancy announcement, an exciting and joyous moment, swiftly transforms into a digital whirlwind of unsolicited advice and unexpected connections.

You post the adorable sonogram or the clever "bun in the oven" reveal, expecting some warm congratulations and a sprinkle of well-wishes. Little did you know, you were about to embark on a virtual journey filled with perplexing advice, YouTube rabbit holes, and the revival of relationships you barely remember.

Within minutes, your social media channels light up like a star-studded concert, with comments and messages flooding in from acquaintances you've long lost touch with. They insist on sending you articles, YouTube links, and unsolicited parenting books that promise to have all the answers. It's like they've been waiting for this moment their entire lives to unleash their troves of parental wisdom.

Intrigued, you click on a few links out of sheer curiosity. After all, who wouldn't want a glimpse into the secret world of parenting hacks? Little did you know that you were about to fall headfirst into the rabbit hole of contradictory advice.

One moment, you're reading an article extolling the virtues of breastfeeding, insisting it's the only way to ensure your child's future success as a rocket scientist. The next, you're watching a YouTube video where a mom swears by formula, claiming her baby sleeps like a hibernating bear. And then there's the unsolicited parenting book that claims both breastfeeding and formula are obsolete because your child should be surviving solely on a diet of kale smoothies and tofu nuggets.

As you wade through this digital sea of contradictions, you can't help but long for the simplicity of the pre-internet era. Back then, you'd rely on your family's advice, your trusted doctor, and maybe a well-worn parenting book that you could hold in your hands, rather than an endless stream of opinions from virtual strangers.

In the end, while the digital age has its perks, it also brings with it an overwhelming tide of information and, often, unsolicited advice. As you close your laptop or put away your smartphone, you can't help but appreciate the value of a personal conversation and the wisdom of your own instincts. Parenthood may be a journey filled with uncertainty, but one thing is clear: the pre-internet era had its own charm.

You're the captain of your pregnancy ship. While you may have a few unsolicited advisors on board, you're ultimately in charge. So, nod and smile, and then continue with your day. And in the future, you might find yourself sharing your own unsolicited advice with a fellow expectant parent, and the cycle shall continue forevermore.

Chapter 7

Symphysis Pubis Dysfunction: A Comedy of Dressing and Distress

Symphysis Pubis Dysfunction (SPD), the cheeky prankster of pregnancy, takes the simple act of getting dressed and turns it into a comedy show that's both painful and, well, anatomically surprising. If you're lucky enough not to experience SPD, I have only one question for you: How does it feel to be God's favorite?

Let's set the scene: You're standing there, clothes in hand, ready to embark on the grand adventure of dressing yourself. Your pelvis, under the mischievous influence of SPD, chuckles ominously, like a cartoon villain hatching a plot.

As you attempt to put on your pants, it's as if your body sends out distress signals to your nether regions. It's like your lady bits have suddenly been elected the unofficial spokesperson for your entire pelvic region, and they're not thrilled about the job.

Each leg you lift into your huge tighty whities, which have somehow evilly replaced your sexy lace thong, feels like a negotiation between stubborn mules, tearing each other in opposite directions. The pelvic bone, always a dramatic bitch, decides to throw in a surprise cameo—a sharp pain right smack dab between your legs, just to keep things interesting. You cry out a colorful string of cuss words that would make a sailor blush.

So, here's to mastering the art of getting dressed during pregnancy, one burning va-jay-jay at a time!

Chapter 8

Parenting Prep: Adventures in Baby Furniture and Birth Playlists

Preparing for parenthood is a bit like embarking on a quest to assemble the most complicated piece of IKEA furniture while also curating the ultimate birth playlist. It's a comedic balancing act of confusion, anticipation, and perhaps a touch of delusion.

Baby Furniture: Not Just Adult LEGO

The crib - the first piece of furniture your baby will call home. It's meant to be a symbol of comfort and safety—a place where your little one will dream sweet dreams of milk and cuddles. But as you embark on the great crib assembly adventure, you quickly discover that it's more of a journey through a labyrinth of confusion and frustration.

Armed with a box of seemingly unrelated wooden pieces and an instruction manual that reads like a foreign language translation gone wrong, you and your partner dive headfirst into the assembly process. The promise of providing your baby with a cozy sleep haven drives you forward, but it doesn't take long for the reality of the situation to set in.

The first hiccup occurs within minutes of opening the box. You find yourself holding a mysterious wooden widget that looks like it belongs to an entirely different piece of furniture.

You glance at the manual, then back at the widget, and back to the manual again. It's a conundrum. You're convinced that this widget serves some critical purpose, but where it belongs remains a mystery.

Three hours into the ordeal, you're both starting to feel the strain. Frustration mounts as you discover that a few of the screws are missing and that the allen wrench provided appears to have been designed for a leprechaun. It's around this time that the first argument erupts. Was it really necessary to embark on this DIY crib adventure? Couldn't you have just bought one pre-assembled?

But you persevere, convinced that you can conquer this challenge. Two hours later, you finally stand back and admire your handiwork. It's beautiful and a testament to your determination and teamwork. You feel a sense of pride welling up as you picture your baby sleeping soundly in this perfectly crafted crib.

Then the revelation hits you like a ton of building blocks. You've put the side rail on backward. In your eagerness and exhaustion, you've made a crucial error that has turned your beautiful crib into a potential safety hazard. You're left with no choice but to dismantle a significant portion of your creation, all while grumbling and cursing under your breath.

Finally, after much trial and error and maybe a call to the friendly folks at customer service who guide you through your predicament, the crib is complete. It may not be perfect, and it may have a few dents and scratches from your assembly escapades, but it's ready for your baby's arrival.

Changing Tables and Gravity

After conquering the crib, you turn your attention to assembling the changing table. This time, you're feeling pretty confident. You've already conquered the crib, after all. What could go wrong with a simple changing table?

As you carefully follow the instructions, attaching legs, securing shelves, and tightening screws, you begin to feel a sense of accomplishment. The changing table starts to take shape before your eyes, and you can already envision the countless diaper changes and baby giggles that will take place here.

With the final piece in place, you step back to admire your handiwork. The changing table is sturdy, functional, and looks pretty darn good, if you do say so yourself. You pat yourself on the back for a job well done.

But then comes the moment of truth. You place a diaper on the table, and as if guided by some mischievous force of nature, it starts to slide slowly toward the edge. You watch in disbelief as gravity asserts its dominance over your changing table. The diaper inches closer and closer to the edge, as if daring you to defy the laws of physics.

With a sigh, you realize that it's time to revisit those f@*k!ng instructions.

The Quest for the Perfect Birth Playlist: DJing for a Tiny Audience

Now, onto the birth playlist, the soundtrack to your baby's grand entrance into the world. You meticulously curate a list of songs that are equal parts soothing and motivational. You consult friends and family for their input, secretly hoping that your baby will appreciate your impeccable taste in music.

You spend hours deliberating over the order of songs, envisioning the perfect musical journey for your little one. You start with calming melodies and gradually build to epic anthems for that triumphant moment of birth. You even throw in a few tracks for your partner, who doesn't quite understand why "Eye of the Tiger" is a birthing necessity.

But as you're deep into the playlist-making process, reality strikes: you've been overthinking it. You realize that your baby will neither judge nor appreciate your carefully crafted playlist. In fact, they might just decide to make their debut during the first track, throwing your entire musical agenda into disarray. (But let's be real, it probably won't be the first track, so maybe don't bet the farm on that.)

53

Chapter 9

Body Changes: When Your Body Forgets It's Not a Theme Park

Pregnancy brings a myriad of body changes: some awe-inspiring and others downright rude. In this chapter, we'll explore the journey of realizing you haven't seen your lady parts in weeks and you're not, in fact, glowing; you're sweating.

Where's My Vag? The Vanishing Act

Somewhere around the midway point of your pregnancy, you glance down and suddenly realize you haven't seen your own vagina in weeks. It's become an elusive little creature, hiding beneath the ever-expanding bump that now occupies your personal space. It's almost like it's gone on vacation without leaving a forwarding address.

You attempt a daring expedition, bending forward in an attempt to make visual contact. But alas, all you see is a charming view of your burgeoning belly, and you get even more lightheaded in the process. You chuckle at the absurdity of it all, wondering if there's a "Missing 'gina" poster you should be putting up around the house. I'm sure your partner would be more than keen to aid in the search.

Boobies: The Overenthusiastic Water Balloons

Remember those days when your bras fit like a charm? You could toss on any top, and your boobs stayed put, just hanging out and minding their own business. Well, prepare yourself for a wild ride because those days are long gone. Your breasts have now taken on a life of their own, and they've enrolled in the School of Overzealous Body Changes.

Firstly, they've decided it's time to grow. Not just a subtle, polite growth spurt, mind you, but a full-on, "hold my drink while I expand to uncharted territories" type of growth. You might wake up one morning and realize you've got cleavage for days, the kind you previously reserved for Victoria's Secret models. Suddenly, the entire upper half of your wardrobe is off-limits. Remember that button-up blouse you used to love? Yeah, that's not happening anymore. It's now the great boob battle to see whether the buttons will stay closed or pop open like a champagne cork at a New Year's Eve party. Champagne you won't be enjoying, albeit.

But it's not just the impressive growth that'll leave you baffled; it's the tenderness. Your boobs will become more sensitive than a high-strung diva on a movie set. A mere graze from your partner's arm will send you yelping in pain, clutching your chest like you've been struck by a medieval arrow. You'll start to wonder if your breasts are training to become the world's next great opera sopranos, with their ability to hit the highest notes of discomfort.

And then there's the leaking. Oh yes, your boobs have decided that they're not content with just growing and aching; they also want to express themselves. In the middle of a romantic movie scene, you might suddenly feel a warm, wet spot spreading across your chest. It's like your nipples have turned into tiny, rebellious fountains, surprising you with their impromptu performances. If your boobs could talk during these moments, they'd probably scream: "Look at us! We're getting ready for the baby!" Yes, thank you, boobs, but could you please be a little less enthusiastic about it?

In conclusion, your pregnancy boobs are like two overenthusiastic water balloons, ready to burst at any moment with growth, tenderness, and surprise leaks. While they may be a handful (literally), they're just one of the many quirky sidekicks on your journey to motherhood. Embrace the chaos, invest in some comfortable bras, and remember that your boobs, for all their quirks, are doing an incredible job getting ready for the newest member of your family.

Bladders with Commitment Issues

Remember the golden days when you could watch a three-hour epic movie without even a hint of bladder-related distress? Ah, the simple pleasures of life! Well, buckle up because you're about to embark on a bladder-related adventure that's more thrilling than a suspenseful movie plot. Welcome to the world of Bladders with Commitment Issues!

Your once-predictable bladder has turned into a drama queen with commitment issues – a complete personality overhaul during pregnancy. It's as if it's decided to go on strike, protesting against its previous role as the quiet, dependable member of your bodily team. Now, it's all drama, all the time.

Firstly, your bladder has decided that it's tired of being spacious and accommodating. It's like it went to a minimalist design school and came back as the proud owner of a thimble-sized storage unit. Suddenly, your trips to the bathroom become as frequent as a cat's demand for treats. You'll wake up in the middle of the night, feeling the urgent need to pee, only to discover that you were just there ten minutes ago. You'll start timing your water intake like a military operation, trying to avoid unnecessary pit stops during important meetings or long car rides.

But that's not all! Your baby has taken up soccer in your womb, and your bladder is its favorite target. It's like your little one has a miniature soccer field in there, complete with goalposts made of your bladder walls. Every kick, twist, and turn sends your bladder into a frenzy. It's as if your baby is practicing penalty kicks with your bladder as the ball, and trust us, your bladder is not winning any goalkeeper awards.

The Glowing Oven: When Pregnancy Turns You into a Human Sauna

"You're glowing!" they said, and you basked in the compliments, imagining yourself as a radiant goddess. But what they didn't mention is that this glow comes with a catch: you'll feel like an oven baking a bun at 350°F. Welcome to the world of night sweats, hot flashes, and a perpetual feeling of summer, even in the dead of winter. Say hello to the furnace life!

Pregnancy hormones, those cheeky little tricksters, have decided to turn up the heat, and you're the unsuspecting victim caught in their fiery antics. Suddenly, your body temperature is cranked up to the maximum setting, and it seems like your internal thermostat is stuck on "tropical paradise."

Night sweats become a nightly ritual. You'll wake up in the wee hours of the morning, drenched in sweat, feeling like you've just finished an intense hot yoga session while wearing a winter coat. Your once-beloved cozy pajamas are now a breeding ground for moisture, and your bed sheets could double as a waterpark slide.

Hot flashes? You'll experience them at the most inconvenient moments, like during a work meeting or while grocery shopping. It's like your body is playing a game of "temperature roulette," and you're never quite sure when the heatwave will strike. Your face will turn beet red, and you'll fan yourself with whatever is within arm's reach, whether it's a piece of paper or your partner's hand. It's a bit like having your very own portable sauna experience everywhere you go. Fun, right?

Even in the depths of winter, when everyone else is bundled up in layers of cozy sweaters and scarves, you'll be the one person walking around in a T-shirt and flip-flops, as if you've been transported to a tropical island against your will. Your friends and family will look at you with a mix of sympathy and amusement, wondering how you manage to stay cool (or should we say, hot) under pressure.

The Belly Button: The Unexpected Drama of Naval Affairs

Ah, the belly button. That humble little dimple, which for most of your life has existed as an unobtrusive reminder of your time in the womb. But pregnancy, with its never-ending surprises, has taken it center stage. Suddenly, your navel has grabbed the spotlight, and it's going through more transformations than a character in a telenovela. Who knew you had such a theatrical belly button?

As your belly expands, so does the drama. One morning, as you're inspecting your ever-growing tummy, you'll spot it—the first signs of your belly button's big debut. It's starting to flatten out, moving from the "innie" club to somewhere in between. You might find yourself wondering if it's taking lessons from a pop-up book because just when you think it's done surprising you, it pops out even more.

Now, every piece of tight clothing becomes a stage for your navel's one-person show. Put on a snug shirt, and voilà, there's a little bump where there once was a dimple. Your belly button, in its newfound "outie" glory, seems to wave hello to anyone who happens to glance your way. But don't fret, use this time to give that bad boy the cleaning it deserves.

Chapter 10

Delivery Day Fantasies: Oscar-Worthy Performances and Playlist Nightmares

The days leading up to your due date are a blend of excitement, anxiety, and wild daydreams about what delivery day will be like. In this chapter, we delve into the world of delivery day fantasies, from practicing Oscar-worthy performances to the nightmare of the delivery room playlist gone rogue.

The Birthing Video Marathon: Prepping for Your Close-Up

You find yourself deep in the YouTube rabbit hole, watching birth videos with a mix of fascination and sheer horror. As each video unfolds, you take mental notes: the calm breathing techniques, the whispered affirmations, and the determined gazes of the expectant mothers.

You begin to wonder if you should practice your own Oscar-worthy performance. Should you work on your dramatic pauses and inspirational speeches? Perhaps you should rehearse your best "This is it, my moment of glory" expression in the mirror. After all, you've been preparing for this role for the past nine months.

The Delivery Room Playlist: Carefully Curated, but Beware of "Ring of Fire"

You've spent weeks curating the perfect delivery room playlist. It's a symphony of soothing melodies, empowering anthems, and songs that make you feel like you can conquer the world. You've tested it during late-night drives, imagining the baby's arrival to the sound of soft acoustic guitars and heartfelt lyrics.

But there's a nightmare lurking in the depths of your playlist. It's that one song, the one that doesn't quite fit the serene atmosphere you're aiming for. You're afraid that, in the heat of the moment, your playlist will suddenly shuffle to "Ring of Fire," and you'll find yourself pushing to the rhythm of Mr. Cash, while ironically experiencing that 'ring of fire' yourself.

Embracing the Fantasies
Amid these delivery day fantasies, you come to realize that they're a natural part of the journey and will likely never go as planned. They're a blend of nerves, anticipation, profanities, and the desire to create the perfect atmosphere for your baby's arrival.

Because to the world, you're a mother-to-be. But in the eyes of that little one, looking up at you for the very first time, you are everything.

Go get 'em, Superhero. The real adventure is just beginning.

Epilogue

The Beginning of Forever

Throughout the journey of this book one thing becomes abundantly clear: parenthood is a delightful comedy of errors. We find ourselves at the starting line of a new adventure, the beginning of parenthood. The laughter, the camaraderie, and the shared tales, cravings, body changes, and unexpected delivery room playlist mishaps have paved the way for the grand finale – the arrival of your precious little one. The journey you've embarked upon is a journey of love, where laughter and cuss words are the glue that binds the pages of your unique story. As you hold your baby for the first time, remember that this is just the beginning of a lifetime filled with moments of joy and mirth. The adventures of parenthood may be unpredictable, but they are also a treasure trove of memories that will forever warm your heart. So, with love and laughter as your guides, step boldly into the beautiful chaos of parenthood, for this is the beginning of forever.

About the Author

Julia Duffy is a writer and a mother who has navigated the enchanting yet sometimes perplexing world of pregnancy. Drawing upon her own experiences and the stories of others, she brings you this whimsical and relatable account of the quirks and culinary escapades that come with the territory of expecting a child. With a passion for storytelling and a sprinkle of humor, Julia Duffy invites you to join her on this unique journey.